Teaching Affirmative Consent

Practical Guidelines to Increase Student Understanding

Gina Lepore, MEd

Brittany Louise-Hoffman Lucas, MPH, CHES

Marcia Quackenbush, MS, MFT, MCHES

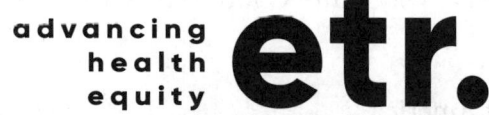

advancing health equity etr.

ETR (Education, Training and Research) is a nonprofit organization committed to providing science-based innovative solutions in health and education designed to achieve transformative change in individuals, families and communities. We invite health professionals, educators and consumers to learn more about our high-quality programs, publications and applied research, evaluation and professional development services by contacting us at 100 Enterprise Way, Suite G300, Scotts Valley, CA 95066, 1-800-321-4407, etr.org.

Published by ETR, 100 Enterprise Way, Suite G300, Scotts Valley, CA 95066-3248

Title No. A534

Printed in the United States of America

ISBN 978-1-56240-172-6

19-0220

Contents

Acknowledgments

We wish to thank the health professionals, researchers, health educators and classroom teachers who reviewed the drafts of this publication and participated in field testing. We appreciate their commitment to providing youth with effective education and meaningful skill-building. Their suggestions have helped us improve this resource.

We dedicate this supplement to them and their important work.

We would especially like to thank:

Al Vernacchio, MSEd, Sexuality Educator, Author, Speaker
    Friends' Central School, Wynnewood, PA

Jacque Hartke, Health Teacher
    Santa Cruz High School, Santa Cruz, CA

Onika Henry, MEd, Sexuality Educator
    Trinidad & Tobago

Shanna M. Dusablon Drone, MSW, MAEd, MAEd, MEd, Sexuality Educator
    Victorville, CA

Michelle Melby, Kurt Nickerson, and Rebecca Oliphant, Teachers,
    James Lick High School, San Jose, CA

We also wish to thank the students who participated in pilots of this lesson plan and provided feedback on the content. Their insights and observations helped us develop a better lesson.

Introduction

Why This Supplement Was Developed

Most of the proven programs addressing pregnancy, STD/HIV prevention and other aspects of sexual and reproductive health were originally designed and tested many years ago. Since then, cultural perspectives, organizational policies and local and national laws have changed. So have some trends in youth behaviors. Social media and Internet resources now play a significant role in informing young people about human sexuality and shaping youth behaviors.

Many of our evidence-based interventions (EBIs) benefit from modest updates that take some of these changes into account. One area where this is true is the matter of Affirmative Consent—the principle that positive and Affirmative Consent ("Yes Means Yes") must be offered by both partners actively and consistently throughout a sexual encounter.

We believe that creating positive norms about Affirmative Consent will play an important role in supporting healthy choices and reducing sexual risks. These standards assert that it is essential for young people both to know their limits in romantic relationships and to understand their own wishes. It is equally necessary that they discover and respect their partner's limits and wishes.

This supplement—which includes background information, a one- or two-session class and a Discussion Guide—was developed to offer educators opportunities to bring Affirmative Consent into lessons about sexual and reproductive health. It is designed to comply with guidelines for allowable adaptations in evidence-based programs. It can also be used with programs that are not considered evidence-based.

6 Good Reasons to Teach About Affirmative Consent

We think teaching about Affirmative Consent is a great idea. Here are some of the reasons why:

1. **It builds communication skills.** The practice of Affirmative Consent requires competence in communication, especially the ability to express one's own wishes and listen to and check in with a partner. This requires attention to both verbal and nonverbal communication, as well as the understanding that nonverbal communication is not always clear. Better communication can also build more satisfying sexual experiences at

whatever point students do become sexually active. Finally, mastering these skills in the context of Affirmative Consent can improve students' general communication abilities.

2. **It offers a positive, respectful frame about personal choice.** Affirmative Consent principles give young people a positive framework for making personal choices about romantic and sexual behaviors. The focus is on respecting personal limits while negotiating what each partner wants, rather than on defensive negotiation or pressure.

3. **It responds to shifting cultural norms.** Increasingly, individuals, organizations and policy bodies are addressing Affirmative Consent and integrating it into educational programs. Many sexuality and health educators now consider an Affirmative Consent perspective essential in effective sexuality education.

4. **It helps prevent sexual assault.** The primary purpose of Affirmative Consent standards is to prevent sexual assault. When both partners in an encounter put Affirmative Consent principles into practice, sexual assault, by definition, cannot occur. Both partners check for and affirm that consent is present. If there is uncertainty or doubt at any time, consent is not present and sexual activity must stop.

   We want young people to expect these standards of themselves and their partners. This can help build norms that encourage youth to leave situations where consent is not being respected, ideally before any assaultive behavior occurs.

5. **It supports law and policy.** In some districts and states, this teaching helps schools and educators comply with laws or policies that require teaching about Affirmative Consent. It also helps inform students about laws and policies in their own communities and schools.

6. **It recognizes new social paradigms and addresses negative gender roles.** Young men are often socialized to believe it is their role to be a sexual aggressor and keep pressuring a partner who seems uncertain or says no. Young women are often socialized that they need to set limits repeatedly— they are responsible for keeping sex from occurring. These messages create norms that suggest males must demand sex in a predatory manner, while females should not have sexual desires.

   When we change these social paradigms through practices such as Affirmative Consent, we create opportunities for positive relationships built on mutual respect. Everyone can say yes, and everyone can say no. We limit the likelihood that sexual assault will occur as the result of misunderstanding, miscommunication or false expectations.

Critiques of Affirmative Consent

There is a robust debate about the value of Affirmative Consent. Critics often describe it as unrealistic and complain that it interferes with the natural spontaneity of sexuality—that it "kills the mood." Some say that women should simply speak up and say No if they don't like what's happening.

It isn't our purpose to respond to all criticisms, but we wanted to share some perspectives from our own experiences as educators and trainers. First and most importantly, we promote Affirmative Consent because it offers an opportunity to improve communication about relationships, intimacy and sexuality.

Couples of all genders and orientations who practice Affirmative Consent often describe it as liberating, bringing more joy and excitement to romantic and sexual encounters. They like knowing that their partner is enjoying the moment. They appreciate the freedom to ask for the attentions they desire. For these individuals, Affirmative Consent has been both realistic and enriching.

It would be ideal if individuals of any gender could say No freely—and be heard. Unfortunately, this does not always happen. In a study among Midwestern college students,[1] for example, men relied more on nonverbal cues to interpret that a partner had given consent for sex, even though these cues are less clear than verbal communication. Other studies (cited in the same article) suggest that men are likely to overinterpret women's interest in sex and see refusal as token, believing that when women say No, they really mean Yes.

People are sometimes unable to speak up and say No because they are frightened or confused, or for other reasons (e.g., inebriation, illness, fatigue). In fact, in a set of testimonials from men who acknowledged pressuring or forcing partners to have sex,[2] their language often indicates they did not notice a partner's negative cues. Indeed, some did not even look in a partner's face during the encounter. However, in some of these instances, once a man became aware of a partner's discontent, he stopped. If these men had learned the basic communication skills required in Affirmative Consent—to *listen* to their partner, *express* their own wishes and *respect* one another's limits—the assaults might not have occurred in the first place.

Despite these challenges, most couples are able to negotiate sex successfully most of the time. In instances where non-consensual sex does occur, however, the consequences are serious, resulting in trauma for those assaulted and sometimes for those who pressure or force as well. This is one of the most

---

1   Jozkowski KN, Peterson ZD, Sanders SA, Dennis B, Reece M (2014). Gender differences in heterosexual college students' conceptualizations and indicators of sexual consent: Implications for contemporary sexual assault prevention education. *Journal of Sex Research* 51(8), 904-916.

2   Baker KJM (2012). Rapists explain themselves on Reddit, and we should listen. *Jezebel*. Accessed 1/27/17 at http://jezebel.com/5929544/rapists-explain-themselves-on-reddit-and-we-should-listen.

important reasons to encourage teens and young adults (and any other sexually active individuals) to learn about and use principles of Affirmative Consent.

How the Supplement Was Developed

ETR is the largest producer and distributor of evidence-based interventions today. Our trainers help schools and educators around the nation implement these programs effectively. Most of the programs include activities where students practice refusal skills—saying no to sexual pressure, then using specific strategies to continue building a relationship or, when appropriate, leave a situation.

These are important skills for students to learn. However, this focus on repeatedly saying No can give the impression that sexual pressure is an expected norm in relationships. Educators in our trainings asked for guidance about this. They wanted to reframe these activities in ways that emphasized mutual respect and Affirmative Consent. We had requests for a classroom session that honored the foundations of existing evidence-based programs while helping students learn about Affirmative Consent.

This supplement is a direct response to these requests. We used the suggestions of many of these educators as we conceptualized and developed these materials. The materials were also reviewed by sexual health education experts and frontline educators from around the country. The class was pilot tested in different settings. We are grateful for the collaborative spirit that has been central to the development of this resource.

What's in the Supplement?

There are 3 components in this supplement:

1. **Background for Educators:** This *Introduction* and the *Background for Educators* offer information about Affirmative Consent and guidance for using the supplement. You can find a list of "Resources for Educators" here as well.

2. **Supplement Class:** *"What Do You Want?" Understanding Affirmative Consent* is a one- to two-session class. It is designed to be taught before a sexual and reproductive health program. It can also be used as a stand-alone class. In the class, students do an activity where they practice both listening and communicating in verbal and nonverbal ways; learn about Affirmative Consent; then work in teams to analyze scenarios and apply what they have learned.

3. **Discussion Guide:** *Learning About Affirmative Consent* offers both general and specific suggestions for integrating discussions about Affirmative Consent into existing sexual health programs. These steps will reinforce learning from the supplement class across an entire course.

How to Use These Materials

We recommend the following sequence:

1. **Train teachers and other staff.** Use an inservice to discuss the value of teaching about Affirmative Consent, go over educators' ideas or concerns and review how to teach the class and use the Discussion Guide.

2. **Teach students foundation facts.** Many sexual health curricula focus specifically on skills and attitudes that help prevent risky behaviors. They may not offer detailed information on foundation facts about reproductive anatomy, physiology and sexual behaviors. ETR's *The Basics of Reproductive Health* offers 1-, 2- and 3-lesson options for reviewing male and female anatomy and physiology that may be used to supplement these curricula.

3. **Teach the Supplement Class.** When possible, we recommend scheduling two sessions for the class, especially if your class length is 45 minutes. Keeping the class to a single session may limit some important conversations. See the Appendix for an outline of a two-session version of the class.

4. **Teach the existing classes in your sexual risk reduction program in the order given in the curriculum.** Use the Discussion Guide in this supplement to reinforce learning about Affirmative Consent.

Is This an Allowable Adaptation?

If you are working with a funding agency, you will need to check with your grantor to determine if use of this supplement is allowable under the terms of your contract. The following information may help you make that determination.

First and foremost, the supplement class is a true pre-lesson that occurs *before* the sexual risk reduction classes. It does not modify the content or sequence of the classes in any way. It does provide a foundation of learning that can strengthen risk reduction messages.

The Discussion Guide suggests enhancements to classroom discussions and activities. However, these enrichments are minor and serve to strengthen the prevention messages and activities.

General Adaptation Guidance: A Guide to Adapting Evidence-Based Sexual Health Curricula, a set of guidelines for adapting evidence-based programs, can be found at ETR's website.[3] The Office of Adolescent Health has also published an online guide, *Adaptations for Evidence-based Teen Pregnancy Prevention Programs.*[4]

These guidelines make a distinction between minor adaptations, which do not significantly alter content, delivery or core components of a program, and major adaptations, which do make significant changes in these areas.

In the OAH document, minor adaptations include adding reflection activities, adding implementation strategies to better engage participants and revising material to ensure cultural relevancy. The minor customizations in this supplement's Discussion Guide are designed to be consistent with this intent.

In the ETR document, Green Light adaptations include updating or customizing reproductive health information, making activities more interactive and tailoring learning activities to youth culture. Again, the spirit of our Discussion Guide is intended to be consistent with these goals.

Our Discussion Guide also suggests framing refusal skill roleplays with a mention of Affirmative Consent. Educators can remind students that when one partner is required to say No repeatedly, Affirmative Consent is not being practiced. After the roleplay, educators can ask students to discuss reasons someone might feel it is okay to pressure a partner. The class might take a moment to repeat the beginning of the roleplay and demonstrate Affirmative Consent principles being used (e.g., respecting the first No).

---

3   Search on *General Adaptation Guidance ETR* or go to www.etr.org/ebi/programs, click on "Other Free Tools" and navigate to "Stage Four: Implement" for a link. You can find specific adaptation guidelines on the program page for each evidence-based program.

4   Search on *Adaptations for Evidence-based Teen Pregnancy Prevention Programs* or go to https://www.hhs.gov/ash/oah/oah-initiatives/teen_pregnancy/training/Assests/adaptations_for_tpp_programs.pdf.

As long as educators present the full refusal skill activity and cover all of the practice opportunities included in the original program, we consider this a Green Light adaptation. However, we encourage you to check with grantors on your projects about whether they find this an acceptable adaptation.

Can I teach this lesson after a sexual health program?

Our general recommendation is to offer this lesson *before* any sexual health program addressing refusal skills. In some instances, however, educators may not have the time to do so beforehand. Others may be required by their grantor to present only the sexual health program being supported, without any pre-class supplements.

Because this lesson works as a stand-alone class, it can also be offered after presenting a sexual health program. Some educators may actually feel this is a better sequence for their students, with Affirmative Consent learning coming after lessons that focus on refusal skills.

Follow School and District Guidelines

As with any sexual health curriculum, principals and teachers must be certain the program concepts, objectives and approach of the supplement are within district guidelines and have the full support of the administration, the school board and parents whose children are enrolled in the class. Parents should receive written notice describing the goals of the broader sexual health curriculum as well as the supplement, be given an opportunity to review the materials if they wish, and be invited to contact the school if they have any questions or wish to request their children be excluded from participating.

Affirmative Consent: Changing Norms

"Everything is about sex except sex. Sex is about power."[1]

This saying brings home an essential truth. When we talk about norms and conventions related to sex and sexual consent, we are often actually talking about norms related to power.

Power to initiate sex. Power to grant access to sex. Power to deny that access.

In Western culture (and some others), males have historically been tasked with the role of sexual asserter—the power to initiate. Females have been assigned the role of sexual gatekeeper—the power to grant or deny access. At the intersection of these roles is sexual consent: the act of granting or denying permission to engage in sexual activity.

In the past, the outcomes of legal cases involving sexual assault or rape often turned on loopholes where a person charged with rape could be found innocent if the person claiming rape failed to utter a clear, unequivocal No. This might be so even if the claimant had passed out and could not speak. Or was too incoherent from substance use (voluntary or forced) to say No. Or too frightened. Or too confused or unsure of what he or she wanted in the first place. Or raised in a culture where saying No is not acceptable, especially for women. Or afraid of hurting the other person's feelings, or of risking violence in response to a No.

More recently, legislation has been introduced in some states with the intent of closing these loopholes. Sexual assault prevention policies at institutions of higher education have also expanded to include language on affirmative consent. These changes have catalyzed a shift in norms about sexual consent, particularly on college campuses. Increasingly, active consent given by both parties must occur regardless of the personal history, current roles or genders of those involved.

---

1   Credited to Oscar Wilde, probably erroneously, but we love it anyway!

Continuing to Promote Positive Norms

Many young people today would challenge the notion that the conventional gender roles mentioned above—sexual asserter, sexual gatekeeper—still apply to them. Among their peers, it is often quite acceptable for females to initiate sex, and for males to decline. Increased acceptance and representation of LGBTQ individuals and experiences have also revised these norms, allowing for an understanding of sexual dynamics that is less constrained by gender roles, gender binaries or sexual orientation.

Yet it is also true that girls are often still shamed for being sexually assertive. Boys are often still encouraged to initiate sex, even if it's not what they really want to do. Further, we continue to hear of girls who are sexually assaulted and blamed, and boys who assault and are absolved. In order for norms related to consent to continue to change, it must become acceptable for everyone to say Yes and for everyone to say No—as they wish, when they wish, regardless of gender or sexual orientation.

We must relieve young men of the pressure to view sex as a means to establish masculinity or dominance. Within such a framework, boys are more likely to view sexual partners as objects, not whole people. Their confidence and self-concept may be influenced by their ability to have sex, even if this is not what they actually want.

Both young men and young women must be given the agency to freely say Yes or No to sex without being concerned about reputation or ability to keep a partner. When we require girls to be gatekeepers instead of active participants, they are likely to view sex as something to deny or endure rather than as something to honor, enjoy and participate in as they choose. This is especially important because the gatekeeper role ascribed to females promotes the notion that girls say No not because they mean it, but because they're "supposed" to; or that No actually means yes; or that girls expect boys to keep pressuring them. This is one of the factors contributing to the myth that false accusations of rape are common.[2]

When we endorse the historic norms, explicitly or implicitly, we set our youth up for sexual and emotional failure as they are just starting on their journeys as sexual beings. What if, instead, we encourage youth to employ authenticity and personal agency to guide their sexual choices, and discourage them from judging others' sexual choices? This has the potential to create a generation that has more genuine, consensual and fulfilling relationships.

---

2 National Sexual Violence Resource Center (2012). False Reporting: Overview. Accessed 2/10/17 at http://www.nsvrc.org/sites/default/files/Publications_NSVRC_Overview_False-Reporting.pdf.

Who Commits Assaults and Rapes?

Exactly who perpetrates rape and sexual assault? Conflicting theories about this make it challenging to know where to focus prevention messages and interventions.

One long-standing theory is that a very small percentage of males (perhaps 6%) commit a substantial majority of rapes. These are severe repeat offenders.[3]

Another theory looks at a more complex possibility. There is data that suggests that some rapists are indeed severe repeat offenders. Others might rape once or twice. There is, additionally, a group that doesn't realize that their approach to sex is harmful, non-consensual and assaultive, and that what they are doing is, in fact, rape.[4,5]

It is also true that some females sexually assault and rape. However, the rates of perpetration by males vastly overshadows those by females.[6,7]

Whichever theory one prefers, one conclusion from the available data is that many young people *do* understand the concept of consent in sexual interactions. Many already ascribe to the norm that "No" means *No* and "Yes" is the only thing that means *Yes*. In all or most of their sexual encounters, these are the principles they put into practice.

Reaching All Students

This is one of the reasons we like the general approach of this lesson. It seeks to reach all students to address misperception of norms about consent. Building this understanding will be helpful for students at risk to commit assault as well as those who are unlikely ever to do so. It will also support those who might be harmed by the disrespect or assaultive behavior of others. Here's why:

- It affirms for young people who already recognize and respect the elements of consent that this is what most of their peers understand and practice, and it is what civil society expects of them.

- It boosts communication skills that can clarify for both partners whether or not consent is present.

---

3   Lisak D, Miller PM (2002). Repeat rape and multiple offending among undetected rapists. *Violence and Victims* 17(1): 73-84. Accessed 2/10/17 at http://www.davidlisak.com/wp-content/uploads/pdf/RepeatRapeinUndetectedRapists.pdf.

4   Thomson-DeVeaux A (2015). What if most campus rapes aren't committed by serial rapists? *FiveThirtyEight*. Accessed 2/10/17 at https://fivethirtyeight.com/features/what-if-most-campus-rapes-arent-committed-by-serial-rapists.

5   Swartout KM, Koss MP, White JW et al (2015). Trajectory analysis of the campus serial rapist assumption. *JAMA Pediatrics* 169(12): 1148-1154. Accessed 2/10/17 at http://jamanetwork.com/journals/jamapediatrics/fullarticle/2375127.

6   National Sexual Violence Resource Center (2015). Statistics about sexual violence. *Info & Stats for Journalists*. Accessed 2/10/17 at http://www.nsvrc.org/sites/default/files/publications_nsvrc_factsheet_media-packet_statistics-about-sexual-violence_0.pdf.

7   Krebs CP, Lindquist CH, Warner TD, et al (2007). The Campus Sexual Assault (CSA) Study. Final report for NIJ Grant No. 2004-WG-BX-0010. Document No. 221153. Accessed 2/10/17 at https://www.ncjrs.gov/pdffiles1/nij/grants/221153.pdf.

- It strengthens the ability and resolve of all young people to look for and insist on respect for these principles.

- It emphasizes that a relationship where personal boundaries and sexual limits are not respected is not healthy.

- It clarifies for individuals who are not currently clear about consent—particularly those at risk to act as perpetrators—that *it is never okay to pressure a person into sexual activity.* It also confirms that the only way to know if a partner consents is to hear a clear *Yes,* both verbally and through body language.

Communication Is Key

Today's shifts in our understanding of consent reinforce that the absence of a clear No does *not* mean Yes. Only "Yes" means Yes. Too drunk to communicate coherently does not mean Yes. Passed out from fatigue or intoxication does not mean Yes. Had sex with one person last week does not mean Yes to someone else this week. Performed oral sex last night does not mean Yes to intercourse tonight. Said Yes to vaginal intercourse then does not mean Yes to anal intercourse now.

How can such clarifications and distinctions be negotiated between two people? Communication. And because in sexual encounters it is easy for people to misunderstand each other and the stakes are so high, more communication is better than less.

Encouraging a shift in our conceptualization of consent and how to communicate about it underscores this undeniable truth: people are better off when both partners involved in sexual activity are engaging with a resounding YES! Why would we want anything different, especially for our youth?

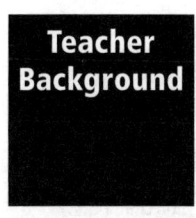

Teaching Affirmative Consent at the Same Time We Teach Refusal Skills

Refusal skill activities teach students how to resist pressure to have unsafe or unwanted sex. They are an essential component of many evidence-based sexual health interventions. Programs that include refusal skills have been found to increase youths' chances of avoiding unwanted sexual pressure. Students receive instruction on the process and then practice delivering effective refusals, such as saying No or suggesting alternative actions.

With greater interest in teaching students about Affirmative Consent, however, many educators struggle with continuing to teach refusal skills. Teachers wonder if repeating refusal skill roleplays and other activities gives students the impression that sexual pressure is normal and to be expected. Some question how they can effectively teach refusal skills and Affirmative Consent side-by-side.

We believe it is not only possible but essential to teach about both refusal skills and Affirmative Consent. The concepts are not mutually exclusive. Both have their value and place in sexual risk reduction interventions.

Refusal skills empower students by giving them a range of effective strategies for resisting unwanted sexual pressure. Affirmative Consent builds students' communication skills and clarifies expectations about respecting each other's boundaries and decisions. When taught together, Affirmative Consent and refusal skills give youth a variety of tools to make healthy choices about sexual behaviors and communicate effectively about boundaries and wishes.

Effective Steps

The following steps can help educators teach refusal skills within the context of learning about Affirmative Consent.

- Make clear to students that if someone needs to say No more than once, that person's boundaries are not being respected. Such situations are not okay.

- Emphasize the importance of refusal skills as a tool for people of any age to respond to unwanted pressure. Saying No effectively in such situations helps people communicate their boundaries.

- Avoid placing responsibility on a refuser to provide a strong No. Be clear that the responsibility is for *both* partners to obtain a clear, unambiguous Yes. Remind students that both parties need to communicate personal feelings and desires while respecting each other's boundaries. No one should ever be pressured. A person who experiences pressure, harassment or assault is not to blame for being the target of these behaviors.

- Use a "bookend" strategy with refusal skill roleplays when possible. First, explain that continued pressure after a refusal or expression of uncertainty is wrong. Acknowledge that students need to learn about refusal skills because in real life situations, people may not always respect limits. Second, do the roleplay as written in the curriculum and discuss as directed. Third, include one or two questions in your debrief about the roleplay that put the focus on the person applying the pressure ("What did the person in the pressuring role say or do to try to convince the other person to change their mind?" "What kind of attitude did the pressuring person have about the other person's boundaries?" "When would it be okay to pressure someone to change their mind after they've said No to sex?"). Fourth, do a quick repeat of the roleplay where Affirmative Consent standards are respected and pressure stops after the first No.

By following these guidelines, educators can continue to teach students refusal skills without contradicting the important messages of Affirmative Consent standards.

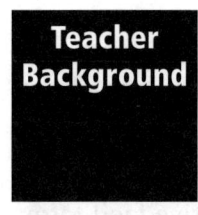

Teaching Affirmative Consent: Assessing and Building Comfort

How do we best teach content areas related to sexuality and sexual health? One of the keys is for educators to assess their own level of comfort with sexual issues, including Affirmative Consent, prior to stepping into the classroom.

Consent can be a sensitive topic. It may bring up more emotions than anticipated, both for educators and students. During conversations about sexual consent, we are likely to see a range of attitudes and misinformation about gender-based norms, sexual scripts, victim blaming and sexual assault. Educators must be able to maintain a safe space for these discussions for all students.

Trauma and Triggers

In any sexual health education program, we must also be mindful of students who may be emotionally triggered by a discussion due to previous experiences, whether or not these were sexual in nature. In matters of consent, students can experience triggers regardless of the role they played—that is, whether they pressured or were pressured, assaulted or were assaulted.

A trigger may transport a student back to the original event (a flashback) or evoke emotions and reactions from that event. Students experiencing triggers might respond in a number of ways during a lesson. For example, they may express strong emotions (e.g., anger, fear, sadness, shame, anxiety), withdraw from participation in the activities, be unable to concentrate or create distractions that disrupt the class.

We encourage all educators in sexual health programs to be aware of trauma-informed educational practices. (See our "Resources for Educators" section to learn more.)

Ready to Respond

This lesson helps students process their own attitudes and assumptions around consent. Educators must be able to recognize and respond to remarks by students that perpetuate and support victim-blaming, gender-based violence and sexual aggression. If a harmful attitude is expressed, an effective facilitator will not simply silence the student. Rather, students will be encouraged to reflect on and understand the consequences (e.g., creating a negative tone in the classroom; normalizing disrespect, pressure, assault; discounting the value of peers; etc.). This requires skill and preparation on the part of educators.

This is why it is so important for educators to be aware of their own attitudes related to sexual consent. Without that awareness, an educator might unintentionally support negative attitudes that place the burden of responsibility on the person being pressured. Unexamined gender role attitudes may also lead an educator to endorse familiar norms that support males as sexual aggressors and females as sexual gatekeepers. They might discount or minimize the possibility of sexual aggression in same-gender relationships.

Navigate Successfully

The following steps can help educators navigate conversations about consent successfully.

- Maintain group agreements (groundrules) throughout the lesson and conversation.

- Ensure that students feel supported to express their thoughts freely. Guide them to do so respectfully.

- Address harmful statements immediately in a manner that increases student understanding of the potential harm of the remark. The goal is reflection and awareness rather than punishment or shame.

- Make appropriate accommodations for students who are triggered and encourage them to participate in a way that is comfortable for them.

- Refrain from any disclosure of personal experiences involving non-consensual sexual activities. This includes stories about family, friends or acquaintances ("people I know").

Are You Ready? Tips for Self-Assessment

Ask yourself the following questions. Consider how your responses may influence your ability to facilitate this lesson plan and conversations about consent. Check the "Resources for Educators" page for readings to help build understanding in these areas.

- *Do I have a solid understanding of current knowledge about sexual assault and violence prevention?* This knowledge will enable you to effectively respond to the "teachable moments" that may arise in the classroom. Reading up on sexism in its various forms (e.g., benevolent sexism, victim-blaming, rape myth attitude acceptance) can help you build your understanding of the foundations of gender-based violence. Sexism is one of its primary underlying dynamics.

- *Am I aware of my own biases around sexual assault and consent? How might these shape my teaching on the topic of consent?* Watch for comments that unintentionally blame a victim, norm the use of pressure tactics, or suggest it's "normal" and expected for young men to pressure partners about sex.

- *When I hear of a situation involving sexual assault, harassment or non-consensual sex, do I have a tendency to "choose sides"? If so, am I more likely to side with the accused or the accuser?* Taking sides is a natural reaction if you, your family or friends have had personal experiences where there were disagreements about whether consent was present. Notice how this tendency influences your attitudes about different elements in the discussions about consent.

- *Will presenting this lesson plan be challenging for me?* The lesson content may raise personal issues. Spend some time reflecting on the strategies you will employ to maintain boundaries between personal feelings and effective facilitation.

The Nature of the Work

The issues raised in teaching about Affirmative Consent may bring distinctive nuances to sexuality education. It is important to remember, however, that there isn't anything new here for sexual health educators. We must always be prepared to respond to negative or harmful remarks, no matter what the topic. We always want to create an open and respectful learning environment. We want to bring sensitivity to the issues facing students who have experienced trauma. And we want to be aware of the ways our own attitudes and experiences might shape our teaching, especially if the consequences might perpetuate harmful myths or stereotypes.

We believe educators who have successfully presented sexual health programs in the past will work skillfully with the Affirmative Consent lesson and Discussion Guide. One of the most encouraging qualities among educators in this arena is their interest in quality improvement. We hope these suggestions and resources will be of use.

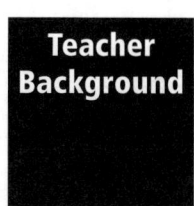

Resources for Educators

Support for Students

Love is Respect. This organization offers 24/7 support and information. People can chat at the website, call by phone at 1-866-331-9474 or text LOVEIS to 22522. www.loveisrespect.org

Trauma-informed educational practices

Use Trauma-Informed Strategies to Transform Your School. An article on the ETR Blog by Alicia Rozum, MSW, PPSC. www.etr.org/blog/my-take-trauma-informed

Helping Traumatized Children Learn. Resource on the Trauma and Learning Policy Initiative (TLPI) website. https://traumasensitiveschools.org

Current knowledge about sex assault and violence prevention

Sexual Violence: Prevention Strategies. Information at the website of the Centers for Disease Control and Prevention (CDC). www.cdc.gov/violenceprevention/sexualviolence/prevention.html

National Sexual Violence Resource Center (NSVRC). www.nsvrc.org

Myths and truths about sexual assault and consent

Sexual Assault Misconceptions. Resource from the University of Michigan Sexual Assault Prevention and Awareness Center. https://sapac.umich.edu/article/52

Gender roles and expectations

In Their Words: How Children Are Affected by Gender Issues. Article in National Geographic by Eve Conant. www.nationalgeographic.com/magazine/2017/01/children-explain-how-gender-affects-their-lives

Gender and Gender Identity. Resource page at the website of Planned Parenthood. www.plannedparenthood.org/learn/sexual-orientation-gender/gender-gender-identity

Teen dating violence prevention

Understanding Teen Dating Violence. Fact Sheet from the Centers for Disease Control and Prevention (CDC). www.cdc.gov/violenceprevention/pdf/teen-dating-violence-factsheet-a.pdf

Teen Dating Violence. More background information from the CDC. www.cdc.gov/features/datingviolence

Teen Dating Violence Prevention Programs. Links to some of the educational programs designed to stop teen dating violence, hosted by the Youth.gov website. http://youth.gov/youth-topics/teen-dating-violence/prevention

Optional Student Resource

Drivers' Ed for the Sexual Superhighway: Navigating Consent. An article by Heather Corinna at the *Scarleteen* website. www.scarleteen.com/article/abuse_assault/drivers_ed_for_the_sexual_superhighway_navigating_consent

Note: Educator review advised. This article offers in-depth, youth-focused information about consent. The language and content may not be appropriate for all students.

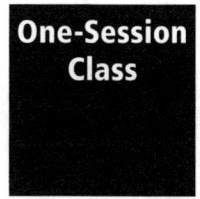

One-Session Class

"What Do You Want?" Understanding Affirmative Consent

Note to the Teacher

This class was designed as either a stand-alone health education activity or a supplement to sexual risk reduction curricula for youth. Ideally, this class will be taught after students have received foundation facts about anatomy, physiology and sexual behavior, and before the classes in the sexual risk reduction curriculum.

As a supplement, the class is designed to create a foundation for discussion about Affirmative Consent throughout all lessons. The class and Discussion Guide provide opportunities for students to understand Affirmative Consent and practice applying its principles in situations similar to those they may face in their own lives.

Trigger warning: *As with any class that addresses issues such as sexuality and consent, students with experience of trauma may find some of the material challenging. We suggest that before the segment "Looking At Stories: Is This Consent?" you state that some of the content may be sensitive for some individuals. Remind students that we all have different experiences, and that it's important for everyone in the classroom to remember and respect this. Some students may have known someone who has been pressured or sexually assaulted. Be available to answer any questions or offer support after the class. There is contact information for a 24/7 hotline, chat and text referral service in both the "Resources for Educators" (p. 11) and "Resources for Students" (p. 38) sections.*

Adapting to a Two-Session Class

We recommend teaching the class over two sessions if possible. In the first session, complete "Let's Have Pizza" and "Definitions: Affirmative Consent." In the second session, have students work in teams to complete the "Looking at Stories: Is This Consent?" activity as written. Then ask teams to write their own pairs of scenarios, one showing consent, the other showing no consent or "Unclear." Have teams share and discuss their scenarios with the full class as time allows. Provide guidelines as appropriate (e.g., no sexually explicit scenarios).

For an example schedule for the two-session version of this class, see the Appendix "Outline for a Two-Session Version of the Class," on p. 53.

Synopsis

In this class, students start with a pair activity in which they practice listening and communicating in verbal and nonverbal ways. They discuss how important it is to both speak up and listen, then talk about how important communication is in pressure situations. They review and discuss a definition of Affirmative Consent. Then they work in teams to apply the things they have learned by analyzing scenarios where consent may or may not be present. The full class reviews and discusses the scenarios.

Goal

To increase students' understanding of what Affirmative Consent means and how to apply that understanding in real-life situations.

Objectives

After completing this supplement class, students will be able to:

- Define Affirmative Consent

- Identify verbal and nonverbal cues that communicate others' feelings, wishes and boundaries

- Distinguish between situations when Affirmative Consent is and is not present

- Apply critical thinking and communication skills related to Affirmative Consent

Key Messages

- All individuals have the right to choose their own likes and dislikes.

- It is the shared responsibility of all parties to obtain Affirmative Consent from partners and respect partners' boundaries.

- Consent can be expressed verbally or nonverbally. Verbal communication should be used to clarify when a situation is unclear.

- Affirmative Consent involves these steps: people listen to one another's words and body language, express what they like and how they feel, and respect and observe one another's boundaries.

Preparation and Materials

▸ Review the **Scenario Card Sets** (Handout S.4) and choose the most appropriate sets for your students.

▸ Make slide or chart paper for **Game Instructions: Let's Have Pizza!** (Slide S.1).

▸ Make slide or chart paper for **Definition of Affirmative Consent** (Slide S.2).

▸ Prepare chart paper for **Language of Consent/Benefits of Affirmative Consent** (Teacher Page S.3). Have markers for student teams.

Hang the pieces of paper around the room before the class with the bottom taped up to hide the content, or plan to have students help you post the pieces of chart paper as you start the activity.

Note: As an alternative, you can create and label 6 columns on a large dry erase board and have students come up to the board to write their answers.

▸ Make **Scenario Card Sets** (Handout S.4), one set for each team. Copy the scenario sets, cut each set into two sheets, then clip the sheets so they stay together as a set. This ensures that each team gets one Consent and one No Consent or Unsure scenario to analyze.

▸ Copy **Resources for Students** (Handout S.5), one for each student.

Note: Be sure to check the listed resources to ensure they are appropriate for your students.

Outline of Activities: One-Session Class

Activity	Time	Materials
Let's Have Pizza!	15 min.	☐ **Game Instructions: Let's Have Pizza!** (Slide S.1), on slide or chart paper
Definitions: Affirmative Consent	15–20 min.	☐ **Definition of Affirmative Consent** (Slide S.2) on slide or chart paper ☐ Prepared chart paper for **Language of Consent/Benefits of Affirmative Consent** (Teacher Page S.3) ☐ Markers for student teams.
Looking at Stories: Is This Consent?	15–20 min.	☐ **Scenario Card Sets** (Handout S.4), one set per student team ☐ **Resources for Students** (Handout S.5), one per student

Note: For an example schedule for the two-session version of this class, see the Appendix "Outline for a Two-Session Version of the Class," on p. 53.

Activities

Introduce Class

1. Describe class. Tell students the class will be doing some activities today that help them look at the ways people communicate. This will include how we express ourselves to others, and how we listen to and understand what others communicate to us. Later in the lesson, the class will talk about some ways to use these communication skills in romantic relationships.

Let's Have Pizza!

1. Introduce the game. Tell students that the first activity is a game. They'll be working with a partner.

2. Explain the game. Show **Game Instructions: Let's Have Pizza!** (Slide S.1) on slide or chart paper and explain the steps.

- **Your team's goal: Create a pizza you'll both enjoy.** You'll be playing a game where your goal is to create a pizza that both of you will enjoy. That means you have to figure out what your partner likes, and your partner has to figure out what you like.

- **Take turns asking yes-or-no questions.** You'll take turns asking each other yes-or-no questions to figure out how you'd like the pizza prepared and what you'd like on it. First one of you will ask 5–7 questions, then the other will ask 5–7 questions.

- **Ask verbally.** You ask your questions *verbally*.

- **Reply nonverbally.** Here's what's tricky. You have to respond nonverbally, using only your hands and your eyes. You won't be using standard nonverbal communication, such as nodding or shaking your head, smiling or frowning, or giving a thumbs up or thumbs down. Instead, you come up with two gestures you make up—one will mean Yes, one will mean No.

  To give the game some challenge, I'd like you to think of non-obvious signals. For instance, you might touch one side of your nose for yes and the other side for no.

- **If you get stuck, you can start over.** If you feel frustrated at some point, work with your partner to find a solution. Your goal is to work together, not against each other. You don't want to trick your partner, but you do want to see what it's like to try to understand some new nonverbal ways to communicate. If you get stuck, you can always start over. Remember—laughter is okay!

Suggest students ask questions that invite new possibilities. For example, in addition to, "Do you like pepperoni?" they might ask, "Are you willing to try kale?"

Answer questions about the activity and clarify instructions as necessary.

Note to the Teacher

Instruct students not to use any inappropriate hand gestures. Most youth enjoy pizza and play the game willingly. If a student is adamant about not liking pizza, you can offer an alternative (salad, sub sandwich, burrito, etc.).

3. **Start the activity.** Break students into pairs. Remind them that one member of the team goes first, with 5–7 questions. Then they trade roles. Let students know that they'll have 3–4 minutes total during which both partners should ask their questions. Monitor the pairs and provide guidance as needed.

4. **Discuss and debrief.** After a few minutes, or as pairs wind down, bring attention back to the full class. Ask:

- How did this go? Is anyone excited about the pizza you're going to order?

Ask a few pairs to describe their pizzas. Notice whether a pair is in agreement about their pizza or whether there has been some miscommunication along the way.

- What was challenging?

Affirm that nonverbal communication may not be easy to understand.

- What did teams do when things became difficult or confusing? (Did any team stop and start over? Was the second time different? How?)

5. **Clarify and link the game to concepts about consent.** State:

- There are many different situations where people might use some nonverbal communication. One is in romantic or sexual situations. Our discussion about the pizza game can also offer us things to think about in romantic situations—especially where partners are communicating and making choices about sex.

  It is very important in these situations to speak up about what you want, and to listen to a partner's verbal and nonverbal communication.

6. **Discuss pressure.** State:

- We've just done an activity that looked at ways to communicate to come up with a plan that worked for both people —in this case, ordering a pizza. You probably did some negotiating or compromising along the way, and hopefully both partners got a pizza they liked.

Ask:

- Can any of you think of a time when you were with a friend or romantic partner and didn't work on negotiating or compromising about an activity—a time when maybe you went along and did something you didn't want to do?

  You don't need to say what happened. But I'm wondering if anyone can say something about what it felt like to be in that kind of situation.

  Look for and affirm answers such as:

  – Uncomfortable

  – Not respected

  – Like maybe I'd made a mistake

  – Frustrated that we didn't communicate better

State:

- So it sounds like we agree that people don't like being pressured to do something they really do not want to do.

Ask:

- Why do you suppose people might go along with something they don't want to do?

  Look for and affirm answers such as:

  – Sometimes people aren't sure how to speak up about their limits.

  – The other person might be more assertive, or less likely to listen.

  – They don't want to hurt someone's feelings.

– They want to avoid conflict.

– They are fearful of losing a friend or partner.

Ask:

- Why do you suppose others might pressure someone?

  Look for and affirm answers such as:

  – They have trouble understanding, listening or respecting limits.

  – They're used to getting their own way.

  – They think that's what they're supposed to do, or that it's okay to do it.

  – They feel entitled or that it is expected.

7. **Review learning.** Ask students:

   - What are some of the things we've learned from the pizza activity and our discussion?

     Look for and affirm answers such as:

     – Nonverbal communication may not be easy to understand.

     – People don't like being pressured to do something they really do not want to do.

     – Sometimes people aren't sure how to speak up about their limits.

     – It's important to speak up about what you want and to listen to a partner's verbal and nonverbal communication.

Definitions: Affirmative Consent

1. **Check student knowledge.** Ask students to think about the term "Affirmative Consent," which is sometimes also called "Yes Means Yes." Ask them to turn to a partner and talk for a moment about what they believe these terms mean.

   After a moment, bring attention back to the full group. Tell students you're going to review a definition of these terms that they'll be using in the next activity. Let them know this definition takes some of the principles from the pizza game and puts them into a definition about making choices and agreements about having sex.

2. **Review definition.** Show the **Definition of Affirmative Consent** (Slide S.2) on a slide or chart paper. Read it through (or have a student read it). Link elements of this definition to the ideas students shared about the meaning of Affirmative Consent.

Affirmative Consent: Yes Means Yes

Affirmative Consent means that both people clearly and freely agree to engage in sexual activity. They have to be awake, aware and able to make decisions. Consent can be given through words or actions, as long as those words or actions clearly communicate willingness and permission. Consent must be ongoing and can be withdrawn at any time.

Note to the Teacher

States, schools and other institutions may have their own definitions of Affirmative Consent that include additional points or otherwise vary from this definition. Be sure to check relevant policies and laws for your setting and adapt this definition to them as necessary.

3. Clarify definition with examples. Emphasize the importance of consent being "clearly and freely given." Ask:

- Can you think of any situations where someone might not be able to give consent?

   Look for and affirm responses that reflect the following situations. Ask as necessary to check for understanding:

- If someone is asleep, can that person give consent for sexual activity? (No, they cannot.)

- What if one or both people are impaired due to alcohol or drug use? Can they give consent for sexual activity? (No, they cannot.)

Note to the Teacher

Issues related to consent and drinking are sometimes unclear. If appropriate for your students, you may wish to clarify that one drink may not leave a person too impaired to make a clear decision. However, when people continue drinking, or when that one drink is large or very strong, or the person is not used to drinking, clear thinking and true consent may not be possible. Remind them that any level of drinking is illegal for people under 21 and specific legal issues may come up when a minor has been drinking and there are questions about consent.

- What if someone is confused or unable to understand what's happening for any reason—language differences, illness, learning differences? Can that person give consent for sexual activity? (No, they cannot.)

- If someone hasn't said No, can a partner assume that means Yes? (No. The absence of a No does not mean Yes.)

- What if someone is being pressured or feels threatened in some way? (No, they cannot give consent.)

4. **Apply to previous learning.** Link this exercise to the pair activity. Say:

- In the pizza game you just played, you were practicing a form of non-sexual Affirmative Consent. You practiced communicating both verbally and nonverbally about your likes and dislikes. In romantic and sexual relationships, people also communicate both verbally and nonverbally about what they want and about their limits or boundaries. It's important for both partners to pay attention to both verbal and nonverbal communication.

5. **Discuss the language of consent.** Tell students that language that says consent is or is not present can be simple. Point out the pieces of chart paper posted around the room. Say:

- Let's do a chart walk. Find a partner and pick up a marker. As a team, move around the room and answer questions on at least three of these pieces of chart paper. (Point to the appropriate pieces of chart paper as you describe their task.)

   What are some ways a person can say No, either nonverbally or verbally?

   What are some ways a person can say Yes, either nonverbally or verbally?

   What can someone say to check if consent is present?

   What are some of the benefits of using Affirmative Consent?

Get teams up and moving. Monitor and offer assistance or suggestions as necessary. After a few minutes, have students return to their seats. Review the suggestions on the pieces of chart paper.

Look for and affirm answers such as the following. Be sure to review any points below for "Benefits of Affirmative Consent" that are not mentioned by students:

Nonverbal No	Verbal No
– Pushing away	– "Not now"
– Avoiding eye contact	– "I'm not sure…"
– Crossing arms	– "I don't think…"
– Turning body away	– "Wait"
– Not reciprocating	– "I like this, but…"
– Silence	– "Please stop"

Nonverbal Yes	Verbal Yes
– Making eye contact	– "That feels good"
– Reciprocating	– "I like…"
– Pulling a partner closer	– "Mmmmm"
– Smiling	– "Yes!

Ways to check for consent verbally

– "Is this okay?"

– "Is that a yes?"

– "Can we try…"

– "I really like this. Do you?"

Benefits of Affirmative Consent

– Build intimacy, enjoyment and trust in a relationship

– Help both partners be "on the same page" and share the pleasure of being close

– Get to know one another and share your likes and dislikes

– Act with respect and maturity

– Reduce the chance that you'll misunderstand or hurt someone

– Follow rules and laws and avoid trouble

6. Summarize. Say:

• Affirmative Consent standards have been put into place to provide better guidance for people engaging in sexual activity. It makes sure that consent is given—affirmatively—by both people. Affirmative Consent requires a Yes. The absence of a No does not mean Yes.

• Affirmative Consent involves these steps: people *listen* to one another's words and body language, *express* what they like and how they feel, and *respect* and observe one another's boundaries.

Write these three words out on a board or chart paper (Listen-Express-Respect) and repeat them.

Looking at Stories: Is This Consent?

Note to the Teacher

Some of these scenarios involve names that are obviously opposite-sex partners, some involve same-sex partners, and many use gender-neutral names. Be sure to check on students' assumptions about gender in the stories. Use their impressions to explore their expectations about male and female roles in negotiating sexual consent.

1. **Describe activity.** Tell students they're going to work together in teams to examine a few scenarios. They'll see if they can agree about whether both people involved have given Affirmative Consent.

2. **Create columns.** Create 3 columns on a board or chart paper. Label columns "Consent," "No Consent" and "Unclear."

3. **Break students into groups.** Each group should receive one set of scenario cards. One will be from the Consent category and one will be from either the No Consent or Unclear categories.

4. **Give instructions.** Ask the students to work together to decide which of the three categories their scenarios belong in.

5. **Full group.** After a few minutes, bring attention back to the full group. Have students put their cards on the board in the columns they selected.

Note to the Teacher

*Refer to **Teacher Notes on Scenarios** (Teacher Key), p. 27. These list each scenario and explain whether or not consent was present and why.*

If you find a card in an incorrect column as you review the cards with the class, ask the full group if they agree with this placement. If they suggest the correct column, move it there. If there is confusion about where the card belongs, place it outside all three columns and say, "Let's come back to this after we've discussed the other scenarios." Students may be clearer about their answers after the discussion of the other scenario cards.

In this activity, avoid "blaming the refuser" for not giving an effective No. One of the essential points of Affirmative Consent is that both partners must receive a clear Yes before engaging in sex. Emphasize that while it's important for everyone to communicate clearly about interests and limits (saying "yes" or "no," for example), it is also everyone's responsibility to understand clearly what a partner wants. In all circumstances, the absence of a clear, freely given Yes means consent is not present.

6. **Review "Consent" scenarios.** Read the scenario to the full class (or, if you have sufficient time, have a student read the scenario out loud). Ask:

   • How did partners express their Yes?

   Clarify the ways both partners paid attention to verbal and/or nonverbal communication. They only acted when consent was clearly present. (You can move fairly quickly through the Yes scenarios.)

7. **Review "Unclear" scenarios.** Ask questions about what each partner is saying and encourage students to identify where there is a Yes, a No or a Not Clear in each scenario. Remind students that when situations are not clear, it is necessary to stop to get clear consent before proceeding.

Note to the teacher

This is an excellent opportunity to clarify the "myth of mixed messages"—that is, the claim that partners (especially girls) give mixed messages about what they want sexually. Examples:

- *Scenario 3.2, Amber and Marcus: Marcus has said Yes to walking home from school with Amber every day. But when Amber kisses him, his nonverbal expression says, "I'm not sure." Amber must treat that as a No until she can clarify what Marcus wants.*

- *Scenario 6.1, David and Chloe: Chloe says Yes to kissing David, and she says No to David putting his hands under her shirt. She is not giving mixed messages. She is setting personal boundaries.*

- *Scenario 7.2, Dylan and Billie: Billie's wishes are not clear in this scenario. Billie may have said Yes to sitting in the school commons with Dylan. Billie also pulls back, says nothing, gives a small smile (which might signal discomfort, anxiety or fear) and responds without enthusiasm to Dylan's kisses. This is a clear message that Dylan needs to check verbally to see what Billie's wishes are.*

8. **Review "No" scenarios.** In these scenarios, one or both partners did not pay attention to verbal and/or nonverbal communication; OR one or both partners could not give consent for some reason (drunk, sick, asleep); OR one or both acted when consent was not clearly present. Ask:

- Who expressed a No in this scenario? How was the No expressed?

- What could the person doing the pressuring have done differently to respect the No? (If both partners were acting without clear consent, what could they both have done differently?)

9. **Address any cards that were placed incorrectly.** Return to those cards and ask students to describe the expressions of Yes or No in the scenarios. Have students suggest the best placement for those cards.

10. **Students review learning.** Ask students to reflect for a moment on the things the class has discussed and learned today. Ask them to write down three key things they have learned about consent and communication.

After a moment, invite students to share some of the things they wrote down. Look for and affirm answers such as:

- It's important to communicate as clearly as possible about likes and limits. That includes both speaking up and listening.

- Any time a situation is unclear, consent is not present. Partners need to stop and check if things aren't clear.

- Partners need to pay attention to body language and facial expressions as well as words.

11. **Summarize lesson.** Say:

- If and when people choose to have sexual relationships, they always get to choose their own likes and dislikes. Everyone is responsible for giving and getting Affirmative Consent from partners. Remember: Listen-Express-Respect.

12. **Resources.** Pass out **Resources for Students** (Handout S.5). *Reminder:* Check resources to ensure they are appropriate for your students.

Extend the Learning (Optional)

You can use the scenarios and other activities for additional learning. Here are some ideas.

- Ask students to write their own scenarios, either as individual homework or a team project. One scenario should show clear consent, and the other should show no consent or be unclear. Analyze these scenarios as you did those in the lesson. (You may want to set some parameters for your students, such as no sexually explicit scenarios.)

- Distribute additional scenario pairs that were not used in class. As a homework or small group activity, have students describe the ways consent is or is not present.

- Ask students to work in teams to create posters supporting essential messages about Affirmative Consent. Post the completed posters in the classroom or in common areas of the school.

- Ask students (individually or in teams) to complete an analysis of popular media, such as movies, TV shows or music videos. Have them identify five instances of romantic or sexual activity portrayed in media and describe the reasons consent was or was not present.

Teacher Notes on Scenarios

Scenario Set 1

1.1 Pat starts kissing Jordan. Jordan kisses back. They make out. *(Consent: This is a nonverbal Yes.)*

1.2 Deka asks Cam for oral sex. Cam says, "I'm not sure I want to do that." Deka keeps asking, hoping to change Cam's mind. After a few more attempts, Cam says okay. *(No Consent: Deka should have stopped after Cam expressed uncertainty. Repeating the request is a form of pressure.)*

Scenario Set 2

2.1 Jela and Casey met a few days ago. They started texting about going to a party together over the weekend. At the party, they both drink and get a little high. Casey asks if Jela wants to have sex, and Jela agrees. After they start making out, Jela says, "I want to stop." Casey doesn't listen and continues. *(No Consent: Both partners are high and may not be oriented enough to give consent. Once Jela says, "I want to stop," consent has been withdrawn and sexual activity must stop.)*

2.2 James and Michael are walking home from school. James reaches out to hold Michael's hand and asks, "Is this OK?" Michael nods and smiles. *(Consent: Both partners show through verbal and nonverbal communication that they consent.)*

Scenario Set 3

3.1 Grace wants to use a condom to have sex. Daniel says, "But it feels better without a condom. Don't you think we'll be safe without one?" Grace shakes her head. Daniel realizes Grace has a good point. He says, "You're right. We should use a condom." He pulls out a condom and smiles. *(Consent: Grace and Daniel negotiate and both consent verbally to having sex with a condom.)*

3.2 Amber has liked Marcus since the start of the school year. They enjoy walking home from school together every day. It is now January, and she has finally worked up the courage to tell him how she feels. While walking home, she lightly grabs Marcus' arm, turns to him, and kisses him on the lips. Afterwards, she notices he looks confused. She kisses him again. *(Either Unclear or No Consent: Amber hasn't asked, verbally or nonverbally, to kiss Marcus. She is not clear how he reacted to her kiss. She needs to check further before proceeding to be sure consent is present.)*

Scenario Set 4

4.1 Jessie is drunk. Kai is not. Jessie starts making out with Kai. Kai is into this, and they make out until Jessie passes out. After Jessie passes out, Kai continues to do sexual things with Jessie, thinking, "Jessie started it and was really into it, so this is okay." *(No Consent: People who are drunk or high cannot give consent. Someone who is passed out cannot give consent.)*

4.2 Sebastian and Elena have been dating for six months. They have made out a few times. Sebastian wants to take things further. One night, he tells Elena about his feelings. He asks what she wants and what she is comfortable with. She tells him she is ready to do more, but does not want to have intercourse yet. They both agree to explore more and let each other know when they want to stop. *(Consent: Sebastian and Elena have given verbal consent to explore more and agree to respect each other's limits.)*

Scenario Set 5

5.1 Ava and Emily are at a party. They make eye contact from across the room, approach one another and begin dancing. Ava pulls Emily close. Emily smiles and embraces Ava. Later on, they make out. They exchange phone numbers. *(Consent: Ava and Emily show nonverbally that they consent.)*

5.2 Kris and Mateo are going out. They have made out and had oral sex before. One night, Mateo wants Kris to give him oral sex. Kris says "I don't want to." Mateo says, "You've done it before, so what's the big deal?" Kris says, "I just don't want to tonight." Mateo says, "You really confuse me when you keep changing your mind like this. Let's do it!" *(No Consent: Although both have consented to oral sex in the past, Kris is not consenting this time. Mateo should not continue to pressure Kris.)*

Scenario Set 6

6.1 David is at a party and sees Chloe. He knows she has a crush on him. He goes up to her and they start talking. He gets her a drink, and then another. Then they go outside and start to make out, both with excitement. David pulls up Chloe's shirt and starts to remove her bra. Chloe freezes. She pulls his hand away but keeps kissing him. A few minutes later, David tries again. Chloe moves his hand away again. They continue to kiss, and David keeps his hands above Chloe's clothing. *(Either Unclear or No Consent: Both people had been drinking. They may not have been able to give consent. Chloe clearly communicated Yes to David about kissing, and No about pulling up her shirt. This was not a mixed message. David tried again, which he should not have done. After that, he only did activities that Chloe had given consent to.)*

6.2 Kadin and Alex haven't seen each other since they broke up a year ago. They meet at a party and start talking. Alex says, "It's good to see you. I've missed you." Kadin says, "I really want to be with you tonight," and pulls Alex in close. Alex resists for a moment and looks confused. Kadin lets go. Then Alex smiles and reaches out to Kadin, saying, "That would be amazing." *(Consent: Kadin and Alex communicate both verbally and nonverbally about limits and consent. Each only moves forward when mutual consent is clear.)*

Scenario Set 7

7.1 Quinn and Morgan are in college. They have been together for three years and last month they got married. One afternoon at home, they begin kissing. They smile at one another, lay down on the sofa and have sex. They look into one another's eyes often and respond to one another with excitement. They never say a word to each other the entire time. *(Consent. Quinn and Morgan give each other repeated nonverbal messages—smiles, expressions in their eyes, excited responses—that communicate they are both enjoying this encounter. In a newer relationship, verbal checks would be a good idea. In this long-term relationship, Quinn and Morgan have learned to read and trust one another's nonverbal communications.)*

7.2 Dylan and Billie are sitting out in their school commons late one afternoon. The school is deserted. Dylan leans over and kisses Billie for the first time. Billie pulls back, says nothing, but smiles slightly. Dylan kisses Billie several more times. Each time, Billie pulls back, then gives that little smile. Billie doesn't seem to kiss back much. Dylan thinks, "Maybe Billie is just not a very good kisser yet." *(Either Unclear or No Consent. Billie's smile might be a Yes, but it also might be discomfort, fear or reluctance to hurt Dylan's feelings. Dylan needs to check further to see what Billie wants.)*

Game Instructions:
Let's Have Pizza!

Your team's goal:
Create a pizza you'll both enjoy.

1. Take turns asking yes-or-no questions.

2. Ask *verbally*.

3. Reply *nonverbally*, using two gestures you make up. One means YES and one means NO. Use gestures that aren't obvious.

   • No nodding or shaking your head.

   • No thumbs up or thumbs down.

   • No smiles or frowns.

4. If you get stuck, you can start over.

Definition of Affirmative Consent

Affirmative Consent:
Yes Means Yes

Affirmative Consent means that both people clearly and freely agree to engage in sexual activity. They have to be awake, aware and able to make decisions. Consent can be given through words or actions, as long as those words or actions clearly communicate willingness and permission. Consent must be ongoing and can be withdrawn at any time.

Language of Consent/ Benefits of Affirmative Consent

Prepare 6 pieces of chart paper to post around the room. Hang the pieces of paper around the room before the class with the bottom taped up to the top to hide the content, or plan to have students help you post the pieces of chart paper as you start the activity.

Note: As an alternative, you can create and label 6 columns on a large white board and have students come up to the board to write their answers.

Label the chart paper as follows:

1. Say NO Verbally
2. Say NO Nonverbally
3. Say YES Verbally
4. Say YES Nonverbally
5. Ways to Check for Consent Verbally
6. Benefits of Affirmative Consent

Scenario Card Sets

Scenario Set 1

1.1 Pat starts kissing Jordan. Jordan kisses back. They make out.

1.2 Deka asks Cam for oral sex. Cam says, "I'm not sure I want to do that." Deka keeps asking, hoping to change Cam's mind. After a few more attempts, Cam says okay.

Scenario Set 2

2.1 Jela and Casey met a few days ago. They started texting about going to a party together over the weekend. At the party, they both drink and get a little high. Casey asks if Jela wants to have sex, and Jela agrees. After they start making out, Jela says, "I want to stop." Casey doesn't listen and continues.

2.2 James and Michael are walking home from school. James reaches out to hold Michael's hand and asks, "Is this OK?" Michael nods and smiles.

Scenario Set 3

3.1 Grace wants to use a condom to have sex. Daniel says, "But it feels better without a condom. Don't you think we'll be safe without one?" Grace shakes her head. Daniel realizes Grace has a good point. He says, "You're right. We should use a condom." He pulls out a condom and smiles.

3.2 Amber has liked Marcus since the start of the school year. They enjoy walking home from school together every day. It is now January, and she has finally worked up the courage to tell him how she feels. While walking home, she lightly grabs Marcus' arm, turns to him, and kisses him on the lips. Afterwards, she notices he looks confused. She kisses him again.

Scenario Set 4

4.1 Jessie is drunk. Kai is not. Jessie starts making out with Kai. Kai is into this, and they make out until Jessie passes out. After Jessie passes out, Kai continues to do sexual things with Jessie, thinking, "Jessie started it and was really into it, so this is okay."

4.2 Sebastian and Elena have been dating for six months. They have made out a few times. Sebastian wants to take things further. One night, he tells Elena about his feelings. He asks what she wants and what she is comfortable with. She tells him she is ready to do more, but does not want to have intercourse yet. They both agree to explore more and let each other know when they want to stop.

Scenario Set 5

5.1 Ava and Emily are at a party. They make eye contact from across the room, approach one another and begin dancing. Ava pulls Emily close. Emily smiles and embraces Ava. Later on, they make out. They exchange phone numbers.

5.2 Kris and Mateo are going out. They have made out and had oral sex before. One night, Mateo wants Kris to give him oral sex. Kris says "I don't want to." Mateo says, "You've done it before, so what's the big deal?" Kris says, "I just don't want to tonight." Mateo says, "You really confuse me when you keep changing your mind like this. Let's do it!"

Scenario Set 6

6.1 David is at a party and sees Chloe. He knows she has a crush on him. He goes up to her and they start talking. He gets her a drink, and then another. Then they go outside and start to make out, both with excitement. David pulls up Chloe's shirt and starts to remove her bra. Chloe freezes. She pulls his hand away but keeps kissing him. A few minutes later, David tries again. Chloe moves his hand away again. They continue to kiss, and David keeps his hands above Chloe's clothing.

6.2 Kadin and Alex haven't seen each other since they broke up a year ago. They meet at a party and start talking. Alex says, "It's good to see you. I've missed you." Kadin says, "I really want to be with you tonight," and pulls Alex in close. Alex resists for a moment and looks confused. Kadin lets go. Then Alex smiles and reaches out to Kadin, saying, "That would be amazing."

Scenario Set 7

7.1 Quinn and Morgan are in college. They have been together for three years and last month they got married. One afternoon at home, they begin kissing. They smile at one another, lay down on the sofa and have sex. They look into one another's eyes often and respond to one another with excitement. They never say a word to each other the entire time.

7.2 Dylan and Billie are sitting out in their school commons late one afternoon. The school is deserted. Dylan leans over and kisses Billie for the first time. Billie pulls back, says nothing, but smiles slightly. Dylan kisses Billie several more times. Each time, Billie pulls back, then gives that little smile. Billie doesn't seem to kiss back much. Dylan thinks, "Maybe Billie is just not a very good kisser yet."

Resources for Students

Understanding and Ending Dating Abuse

Love is Respect. This organization offers 24/7 support and information. You can chat at the website, phone at 1-866-331-9474 or text LOVEIS to 22522.
   Website: www.loveisrespect.org

That's Not Cool. An interactive website with suggestions for ending digital dating violence. Lots of resources. Check out their "Cool/Not Cool" quiz!
   Website: https://thatsnotcool.com
   Quiz: www.coolnotcoolquiz.org

CDC Fact Sheet: Understanding Teen Dating Violence.
   Link: www.cdc.gov/violenceprevention/pdf/teen-dating-violence-factsheet-a.pdf

More About Consent

Sexual Assault Misconceptions. A list put together by the University of Michigan Sexual Assault Prevention and Awareness Center.
   Link: https://sapac.umich.edu/article/52

Consent. A short article on the website StayTeen about why it is important to understand consent.
   Link: http://stayteen.org/keywords/consent

Learning About Affirmative Consent

Using This Discussion & Activities Guide

Use this Discussion Guide to build student awareness of Affirmative Consent across a range of lessons addressing sexual and reproductive health. The following steps will help you use the Guide effectively.

- **Review the general guidelines.** Look over the "Five General Suggestions for Discussion" section below. These general guidelines can be put into practice with almost all learning activities.

- **Find guidance on specific types of activities.** The Guide offers specific suggestions for different activities. Check these as you prepare for your sexual and reproductive health classes. Make notes in your curriculum as needed.

- **Develop a regular practice.** It isn't necessary to ask every question listed in this Guide. Instead, simply make it a regular practice to check in with students about Affirmative Consent once or twice in a lesson. For example, ask whether Affirmative Consent was used in roleplays, vignettes, videos and so on.

- **Frame roleplays effectively ("bookend").** Bookend refusal skill roleplays with messages about consent. Talk about Affirmative Consent when framing these roleplays. Point out that when one partner is required to say No repeatedly, Affirmative Consent is not being practiced. Remind students that in an ideal world people would always respect each other's limits, and one No would be enough. In real life this doesn't always happen. This is why it is important for students to learn refusal skills.

  When doing refusal skills activities where a No must be repeated, take a moment afterwards to do a second version of the roleplay that demonstrates Affirmative Consent principles in action—respect for the first No.

- **Build the habit.** Similar questions and comments are suggested for similar types of activities. As you integrate these questions and comments into your classes, it will become increasingly easy to enhance your classroom discussions and activities.

- **Remember: it makes a difference.** Offering these enhancements takes only a little effort, but they can have a powerful impact on students' understanding and ability to take steps to protect themselves and respect others.

Five General Suggestions for Discussion

There are five general suggestions that appear repeatedly throughout this Guide. By using these, teachers can enhance students' understanding of consent and encourage them to respect both their own and others' limits.

The Five General Suggestions:

1. Ask questions about whether consent is present, and how to check for it if it's not.

2. Analyze ways to enhance the clarity of consent.

3. Ask questions about gender roles and expectations.

4. Frame refusal skill activities, emphasizing that the first No *should* be respected.

5. Watch for language bias, double standards and "blaming the refuser."

Below are examples of each of these general suggestions, some of the points when it would be appropriate to use them, and why they are helpful.

1. Ask questions about whether consent is present, and how to check for it if it's not.

When	What you can say	Why
Roleplays or other activities where negotiations about sex take place.	• Was consent present here? Why or why not? • Did these individuals *listen* to their partner, *express* their own wishes and *respect* each other's boundaries? • *(If no)* What could these partners do or say to check for consent?	Helps students recognize when Affirmative Consent is or is not present. Reinforces essential concepts about Affirmative Consent. Supports strategies and skills that reinforce the use of Affirmative Consent. Emphasizes that no one should be pressured to have sex in the absence of Affirmative Consent.

2. Analyze ways to enhance the clarity of consent.

When	What you can say	Why
Roleplays or other activities where negotiation about sex takes place.	• How well were these partners listening to one another about their wishes and limits? How well were they speaking up about what they each wanted?	Emphasizes the importance of both listening and speaking up.
	• (If well) So they both know about and practice Affirmative Consent.	Reinforces and norms positive behaviors.
	• (If poorly) What could they say or do to check for consent in this situation?	Builds skills for problem-solving and establishing clear, mutual consent.

3. Ask questions about gender roles and expectations.

When	What you can say	Why
Roleplays or other activities that might reflect gender roles and expectations.	• What are the genders of the people in this roleplay? • Would this interaction look different if their roles were reversed?	Helps students examine and analyze whether they have different expectations for young women and young men.
	• Can young people express consent in similar ways, regardless of their gender? Or are there differences? • Why might someone feel it is okay to pressure someone who has already said No?	Identifies common but damaging gender role stereotypes that can interfere with clear, mutual consent (e.g., young men should keep pressuring, young women must set limits, it's okay for young men to choose to have sex but wrong for young women to do so).

4. Frame refusal skill activities, emphasizing that the first No *should* be respected.

When	What you can say and do	Why
Roleplays or other activities where refusal skills are being practiced.	*Say **before** starting the activity:* • Remember, when one partner is required to say No repeatedly, Affirmative Consent is *not* being practiced. In an ideal world people would always respect each other's limits, and one No, or a hesitation, or a look of confusion, would be enough. In real life this doesn't always happen. This is why it is important for you to learn refusal skills. • Why might someone feel it is okay to pressure someone who has already said No? *Take a moment **after** the activity to repeat with Affirmative Consent principles being practiced (e.g., respecting the first No).*	Avoids norming the use of pressure tactics. Students often do these activities repeatedly in a curriculum, and the repetition can imply that pressure is normal. Focuses on the responsibilities of the person in the pressuring role, corrects misperceptions. Norms appropriate responses to refusals and reinforces that clear, mutual consent is the expected standard of behavior.

5. Watch for language bias, double standards and "blaming the refuser."

When	What you can say and do	Why
Roleplays or other activities where refusal skills are being practiced or discussed.	• When Partner A said No (pulled back, looked confused), how well did Partner B listen to A's verbal and nonverbal communication? • Would this interaction look different if the partners' roles were reversed? *Provide emphasis to the role of the* listener. *While it may be necessary to critique someone practicing refusal skills, avoid blaming the refuser (e.g., instead of, "She should have said No more firmly," say, "Tyra said No once, and that's all she should have to say. But in situations where a partner continues to pressure, it's helpful to understand how to make that No stronger so you can stick to your limits and insist on your right to be respected. How could Tyra make that No stronger?").*	Brings attention to the importance of both partners *listening* to one another's verbal and nonverbal expressions. Addresses double standards and negative gender stereotypes. Emphasizes that both partners have the right to either wish for, or refuse, sexual behaviors. Avoids blaming the refuser.

Specific Suggestions for Classroom Activities

Below are a range of ideas for adaptations that can be used to reinforce principles of Affirmative Consent with the most common types of activities used in reproductive and sexual health curricula. Because each curriculum and each activity is distinct, the suggestions may not be an exact match. Tailor these examples to work with the teaching materials in your programs.

Ideally, attention to issues of consent will be addressed in a natural and comfortable way throughout the classes. For example, the teacher might ask one of the suggested discussion questions once or twice during a class. The continued mention of Affirmative Consent reinforces the importance of the concept and practice.

All of the suggestions below will be easier to offer to students who have completed the supplement class on Affirmative Consent.

Setting up groundrules and class agreements

When	What you can do	Why
Establishing groundrules for class discussions.	Be sure to include an item such as: • We will respect one another and respect personal choices, even when we don't agree.	Sets a foundation for principles of respect and active listening—listening carefully, watching for non-verbal communication and respecting a range of personal choices.

Discussions

When	What you can say	Why
Large- and small-group discussions.	See "Five General Suggestions for Discussion," p. 40. These include: ask questions about whether consent is present; analyze ways to enhance the clarity of consent; ask questions about gender roles and expectations; frame refusal skill activities, emphasizing that the first No should be respected; and watch for language bias, double standards and blaming the refuser. • Did these individuals listen to their partner, express their own wishes and respect each other's boundaries?	Builds student understanding of Affirmative Consent. Builds skills in analyzing situations and taking action to affirm clear, mutual consent. Reinforces norms that Affirmative Consent is the expected standard of behavior. Reinforces essential learning about Affirmative Consent.

Activities examining personal choices about risk

When	What you can say	Why
Activities designed to personalize risks for pregnancy and STD/HIV; activities addressing decision-making skills.	• Was consent present when people made their choices? • Did both partners listen, express their own wishes, and respect one another? • How might the things we've talked about concerning clear, mutual consent play a role in the sorts of choices people make about risks?	Helps students recognize that some risks may be taken in the absence of Affirmative Consent (e.g., because someone is coerced or pressured). Suggests that using principles of Affirmative Consent can help people make better personal choices.

Roleplays (scripted/unscripted)

When	What you can say and do	Why
Roleplays addressing skills such as refusal, negotiation (building agreements), suggesting alternatives, building the relationship, seeking help from a friend, etc.	• Was consent present here? Why or why not? • (If no) What could these partners do or say to check for consent? *Say **before** the activity:* • Remember, when one partner is required to say No repeatedly, Affirmative Consent is not being practiced. In an ideal world people would always respect each other's limits, and one No, or a hesitation, or a look of confusion, would be enough. In real life this doesn't always happen. This is why it is important for you to learn refusal skills.	Helps students recognize when Affirmative Consent is or is not present. Supports strategies and skills that reinforce the use of Affirmative Consent. Emphasizes that no one should be pressured to have sex in the absence of Affirmative Consent.

(continued)

Roleplays (scripted/unscripted) *(continued)*

When	What you can say and do	Why
Roleplays addressing skills such as refusal, negotiation (building agreements), suggesting alternatives, building the relationship, seeking help from a friend, etc.	*Ask questions that address the thoughts, actions and decisions of the person in the pressuring role (e.g., "What did the person in the pressuring role say or do to convince the other person to change their mind?" "What kind of attitude did the pressuring person have about the other person's boundaries?" "When would it be okay to pressure someone to change their mind after they've said No to sex?")*	Focuses on the responsibilities of the person in the pressuring role, corrects misperceptions.
	*Take a moment **after** the activity to repeat with Affirmative Consent principles being practiced (e.g., respecting the first No).*	Norms appropriate responses to refusals and reinforces that clear, mutual consent is the expected standard of behavior.
	While coaching and encouraging students to improve their skills, avoid using language that blames the refuser (e.g., instead of, "She should have said No more firmly," say, "Sofia said No once, and that's all she should have to say. But in situations where a partner continues to pressure, it's helpful to understand how to make that No stronger so you can stick to your limits and insist on your right to be respected. How could Sofia make that No stronger?")	Avoids blaming the refuser.
Student-scripted roleplays (full script or half-scripted)	*Ask students to write versions of their roleplay where consent is clearly demonstrated (e.g., a refusal is offered and immediately respected; a partner makes sure consent is present before proceeding).*	Norms appropriate responses to refusals and reinforces that clear, mutual consent is the expected standard of behavior.

Model roleplay

When	What you can say and do	Why
A teacher or students do a roleplay in front of the class to model negotiation, decision-making, refusal skills, etc.	• Was consent present here? Why or why not? • *(If no)* What could these partners do or say to check for consent? *Say **before** the activity:* • Remember, when one partner is required to say No repeatedly, Affirmative Consent is *not* being practiced. In an ideal world people would always respect each other's limits, and one No, or a hesitation, or a look of confusion, would be enough. In real life this doesn't always happen. This is why it is important for you to learn refusal skills. *Take a moment **after** the activity to repeat with Affirmative Consent principles being practiced (e.g., respecting the first No).*	Helps students recognize when Affirmative Consent is or is not present. Supports strategies and skills that reinforce the use of Affirmative Consent. Emphasizes that no one should be pressured to have sex in the absence of Affirmative Consent. Norms appropriate responses to refusals and reinforces that clear, mutual consent is the expected standard of behavior.

Lessons addressing sexual risk and substance use

When	What you can say	Why
Roleplays or other activities that look at the link between alcohol and other drug use and sexual risk-taking.	• These partners have been drinking or using. Are they able to give clear, mutual consent for sex? • When people have been drinking or using, the risk for non-consensual sex goes up. It is easier for someone to hurt a partner or be hurt themselves. • What are some signs that would say someone who has been drinking or using cannot give clear, mutual consent for sex?	Helps students recognize that alcohol and other drug use may make it impossible for one or both partners to offer clear, mutual consent. Helps students personalize the risks of alcohol or other substance use. Helps students recognize signs that consent is not possible. While these will vary by situation, students should understand that a person who, because of substance use, is confused, frightened, sick, clumsy, sleepy, unusually emotional or impulsive cannot give clear, mutual consent.

Informational lecture

When	What you can do	Why
Any lecture or informational material that addresses abstinence, relationships, sexual behaviors, pregnancy risks, STD risks, or other areas of sexual and reproductive health.	*Check for content that requires clarification concerning consent.* *Avoid language bias.*	Integrates into information-focused learning the understanding and expectation that Affirmative Consent is the expected standard of behavior. Avoids blaming the refuser.

Condom demonstration

When	What you can do	Why
Demonstrating correct steps for condom use.	*Add the step: "Both partners give clear, mutual consent to have sex." While steps vary in different curricula, this would be either the first step, or a very early step, in the process.*	Helps students recognize that in any sexual encounter, having clear, mutual agreement is an essential and early step.

Interview (parent, peer, professional, other)

When	What you can do	Why
Students interview a parent, peer, professional or other individual.	*Check worksheets or question sets for language bias (e.g., blaming the refuser, promoting gender-based stereotypes), adapt as necessary.*	Establishes a foundation of respect and understanding.

Brainstorming

When	What you can say	Why
Students generate brainstorm lists.	*Ask questions or add comments about Affirmative Consent if relevant.*	Reinforces the value of taking Affirmative Consent into consideration.

Carousel (writing on pieces of chart paper posted around the room)

When	What you can say	Why
Students work individually or in small groups to write on a series of chart paper pieces or boards around a room.	*Check and comment on language bias when appropriate.* • Was consent present here? Why or why not? • Do these answers reflect the ideas of "listen, express, respect" in terms of giving and getting consent? • In these answers, are young people expressing consent in similar ways regardless of their gender? Or are there differences?	Helps students recognize when Affirmative Consent is or is not present. Brings attention to three essential steps in Affirmative Consent. Helps students examine and analyze whether they have different expectations for young women and young men.

Games (Jeopardy style, etc.)

When	What you can do	Why
Playing team-style games answering questions or providing facts.	*Reframe or expand on questions when appropriate to address Affirmative Consent and clarify misconceptions (e.g., Are people using Affirmative Consent in this example? Are the ideas of "listen, express, respect" being used in this question?)*	Helps students recognize when Affirmative Consent is or is not present. Emphasizes norms of respectful listening and Affirmative Consent.

Make-a-Choice activities

When	What you can do	Why
Making choices on worksheets or as stand-up activities where students move to different areas of the room. These may be based on myths and facts, personal beliefs, experiences or commitments, or other areas of sexual and reproductive health. (Sometimes called "Forced Choice" activities.)	*Check for and adapt language bias in questions when appropriate. Watch for:* • *Language that does not demonstrate Affirmative Consent.* • *Language that does not reflect the ideas of "listen, express, respect" in reference to giving and getting consent.* • *Examples where young women and young men are portrayed in stereotypical ways concerning consent and sexual choices.*	Avoids norming non-consensual behaviors. Avoids norming non-consensual behaviors. When possible, use teachable moments to affirm standards of Affirmative Consent. To avoid reinforcing double-standards for young women and men.

Watching a video

When	What you can say	Why
Watching videos about sexual risks and choices, relationships, reproductive health, STD prevention, contraception facts, and other areas of sexual and reproductive health.	• Was consent present here? Why or why not? • Do the actions and attitudes of these characters reflect the ideas of "listen, express, respect" in terms of giving and getting consent? • In these stories, are young people using similar ways to express consent regardless of their gender? Or are there differences?	Helps students recognize when Affirmative Consent is or is not present. Brings attention to three essential steps in Affirmative Consent. Helps students examine and analyze whether they have different expectations for young women and young men.

Stories, vignettes, essays, poems, letters, skits, scripts, PSAs, song lyrics (using, writing)

When	What you can say and do	Why
Students read, write, analyze or discuss stories, vignettes, essays, poems or other written material related to sexual and reproductive health (e.g., making choices, choosing abstinence, avoiding STD/HIV or pregnancy, taking risks, setting goals, experiencing consequences, solving problems, seeking or getting support, helping a friend, etc.)	*Watch for and comment on language or examples that express bias.* *See "Five General Suggestions for Discussion," p. 40. These include: ask questions about whether consent is present; analyze ways to enhance the clarity of consent; ask questions about gender roles and expectations; frame refusal skill activities, emphasizing that the first No should be respected; and watch for language bias, blaming the refuser and double standards.* *Ask students to write versions where consent is clearly demonstrated (e.g., a refusal is offered and immediately respected; a partner makes sure consent is present before proceeding)*	Reminds students to analyze writings for the presence or absence of consent. Builds student understanding of Affirmative Consent. Builds skills in analyzing situations and taking action to create clear, mutual consent. Reinforces norms that Affirmative Consent is the expected standard of behavior.

Anonymous question box

When	What you can do	Why
Students place written questions into an anonymous question box.	*Reframe or expand on questions when appropriate to address Affirmative Consent and clarify misconceptions (e.g., Does this question take issues related to Affirmative Consent into consideration? Are the ideas of "listen, express, respect" being used in this question?)*	Helps students recognize when Affirmative Consent is or is not present. Emphasizes norms of respectful listening and Affirmative Consent.

Outline for a Two-Session Version of the Class

Outline of Activities: Two-Session Class
(45–60 minutes each)

Class Session 1		
Activity	**Time**	**Materials**
Let's Have Pizza!	20–25 min.	☐ **Game Instructions: Let's Have Pizza!** (Slide S.1), on slide or chart paper
Definitions: Affirmative Consent	20–30 min.	☐ **Definition of Affirmative Consent** (Slide S.2) on slide or chart paper ☐ Prepared chart paper for **Language of Consent/Benefits of Affirmative Consent** (Teacher Page S.3) ☐ Markers for student teams.
Lesson Summary	5 min.	☐ Students review and reinforce learning about definition of Affirmative Consent, Language of Consent and Benefits of Affirmative Consent.

(continued)

Class Session 2		
Activity	**Time**	**Materials**
Looking at Stories: Is This Consent?	15–20 min.	☐ **Scenario Card Sets** (Handout S.4), one set per student team
Writing Our Own Scenarios	25–35 min.	☐ Student teams complete two scenarios each, one showing consent, one showing no consent or an "Unclear" situation. Offer guidelines as appropriate (e.g., no sexually explicit scenarios). Full class reviews these scenarios as time allows.
Lesson Summary	5 min.	☐ Students review and reinforce learning about analyzing situations for the presence of consent. ☐ **Resources for Students** (Handout S.5), one per student